The 11 Effective Fat Loss Habits

By Adam Lee C.P.T

Contents

Are you looking for that next fat loss tip?...........................3

Your Mindsets
Chapter 1
Taking Control of Your Fitness.......................................8
Chapter 2
How To Keep Your Sanity On Your Fat Loss Journey...............16
Chapter 3
Focus on the Big Wins..22
Chapter 4
Knowing Where You Are...30

Your Workouts
Chapter 5
The Best Bodyweight Exercise.......................................39
Chapter 6
Using The Best Types of Exercises for Fat Loss.........................47
Chapter 7
The Most Crucial Type of Training for Getting Leaner and
Stronger..55
Chapter 8
Cardio That Helps You Burn More Fat................................62

Your Diet
Chapter 9
The Crucial Habit To Build Your Own Diet................................68
Chapter 10 How to Estimate Your Calories
Chapter 11
How To Keep Your Hormone Levels From Slowing Down Your
Fat Loss On A Diet..83
Stacking Your Habits One At A Time.............................90

Are you looking for that next fat loss tip?

Are you looking for that one weird tip or the next evil trick to help you burn lots of fat?

When you're starting your workout program, do you tend to look for shortcuts?

Do you look at one tip after another because you're in such a hurry to lose weight?

Have you ever watched so many videos about weight loss tips and find yourself doing nothing?

You know that feeling of being frustrated because you've accomplished nothing after watching all of them.

It almost feels like you're frazzled because you're trying out so many different things and you end up getting no results right?

So why does this happen?

What is it about these fat loss tips and tricks that fail to help you? I'm willing to bet you're probably starting to wonder if there's something wrong with you.

I personally think that this problem comes down to 2 deeper issues.

First off, some of the people in the fitness industry have managed to fool you into thinking that applying some weird tip here and there is going to help you lose 10-15 lbs. off permanently.

They'll try to get you to believe that there's some kind of magic pill or easy way to get the kind of results that you want. You can find quick ways to lose weight effectively but they will take a lot of effort or drugs depending on your preference.

We live in a world where everything is based on events and everybody is looking for the instant quick fix solution. Transforming your body requires you to go through a process. The truth is that the guys and women that you see on the billboards and magazine ads go through a process of eating right and training right.

This brings us to the next and more important issue-consistency. Consistency and improvement make up the majority of the results that you'll see with your body. You'll find them to be the most challenging part of losing fat and transforming your body and this book aims to solve that problem.

It would be so easy for me to tell you to eat less and exercise more.

I could tell you to go best mode! Mutant mode! Flash the x sign with your arms to make you feel better but what happens after a week or two when the novelty and excitement wear off?

How do you create behaviors that get you to do these things consistently?

Research has shown that more than 90% of the people who go on a diet will eventually regain their weight back or worse. People will usually fall off the wagon after the first few months of dieting and training as they start to see less progress than they've seen before.

To top it off, most people usually use the limited amount of willpower that they have to go on a diet. They'll often find that their willpower alone is very limited and using most of it to go on a diet will give them subpar results at best.

So how do you achieve the kind of consistency so that you can lose fat and keep it off for good?

You create it by forming sustainable and constantly improving habits. And creating any kind of habit starts with having tiny habits that grow over time. This book will help you create habits for your mindset, training and diet to help you lose fat.

In this book, you'll have 3 sections.

The first section covers the habits that you can build to have a better mindset for fat loss. This section will show you some of the most effective and helpful mindsets to help you lose fat permanently. The second section will help you build the foundational habits for your workouts. It covers some of the training habits that you need to develop on your fat loss journey.

The third section will help you build your eating habits. It will show you how to build your own diet from scratch. You'll also learn some of the tricks of the trade to help you avoid unnecessary fat loss plateaus.

How To Use This Book

While I would like you to read this book from cover to cover, I'd rather that you take the time to apply each step until it becomes a part of your daily routine. Start with 1 small habit and stick to it for 3-4 weeks. Over time, you'll have several habits that can help you achieve your fat loss goals. Now let's get started.

Chapter 1

Taking Control of Your Fitness

"But it's not your fault!"

How many times have you heard someone repeat this garbage when you watch those silly fitness infomercials?

This happens to be one of the biggest lies in the fitness industry. Not surprisingly, you'll find a lot of statements like these from those who hawk diet pills and weird fitness gadgets.

If you want to transform the way you look, you have to believe that you are in control of your life especially your fitness and health. In fact, you have to believe in it so immensely that it becomes second nature to you. If you don't, you'll always wonder why you're not getting the results that you want with your body.

Do you ever notice that some people always look for all of these tips and tricks for fitness on youtube and yet they do absolutely nothing after watching those videos? They actually believe that the change they want to see will actually just fall on their lap after watching those fitness videos. In short, their fitness or lack thereof happens to them.

Now you're probably asking, "But I thought you said that our willpower is very limited and what if I can't control what I eat? What if I just happen to do that unconsciously?"

When I was just starting out, one of the most powerful realizations for me was the fact that I was responsible for the situation I was in.

It wasn't about blaming myself so much as realizing that I had a lot of influence on my fitness and health. Whether I was conscious of my habits or not, I was the one at the steering wheel of my fitness and health.

This mindset forms such a crucial role to your success in fat loss that not having it would be a deal-breaker. One of my favorite habits when it comes to taking control of my diet and training was to take a look at the root cause of my choices. It helped me to see which series of actions or habits got me those results.

In psychology, taking responsibility is often called having an internal locus of control. People, who have an internal locus of control believe that they are directly responsible for their situation. Here's what the research from the Institute for the Study of Labor in Bonn Germany states:

"We find strong evidence that those with an internal locus of control eat healthier food, exercise more, smoke less and avoid drinking to excess. Interestingly, these relationships persist even after we account for the extent to which individuals are future-oriented and value their health." [1]

Make no mistake about it. You have the body that you've gotten now not because of just one action but a series of actions or habits and how you've set them up consciously or unconsciously. At the end of the day, you're looking at the conscious and unconscious decisions you've made with your fitness based on how you've set things up.

Did you set things up for failure or success?

Take a look at your diet for instance and look at some of the unhelpful choices that you've made. Do you tend to snack on a lot of junk that you really couldn't care less about when you're watching a football game?

Do you tend to eat a lot of junk when you're emotionally upset or when you've got a lot of things to accomplish for the day?

---

[1]Stefanie Schurer, *Healthy Habits: The Connection Between Diet Exercise and Locus of Control* (IZA, 2012).

Ask yourself why you tend to get these habits and keep on asking why until you get to the root of the problem.

You can do this every month as you evaluate some of your habits. Take out a sheet of paper and summarize some of your bad habits.

If you don't know what they are yet, take a look at some of the results that you've been having. Now ask yourself why you got there in the first place. Once you get your answer, you don't stop digging. Keep asking yourself why until you find the root cause of the problem.

The key to making this habit work for you is honesty. Being brutally honest about your results as well as the root causes will help you figure out some of the unconscious decisions that you've made. Remember that these habits took a long time to build and most of them are things that you don't even do consciously anymore. It has become so automatic that you don't even think twice about doing them.

In my case, I noticed that my diet never really got any kind of momentum because I was eating a lot of junk food and processed carbohydrates.

Working in a pastry shop, I was bound to encounter a lot of pies and cakes. I really couldn't find anything else to eat. As the peak days of the week start to approach, we tend to have a pretty busy schedule and I end up getting stressed about it.

It wasn't even a question of if but when I was going to consume a batch of cheesecake that wasn't done perfectly.

So I decided to set up a snack or a meal that I could bring with me to work so I could replace this habit. In my case, I bought some canned garbanzo beans and some hard boiled eggs. I ended up replacing my habit of consuming high calorie foods when I'm stressed.

Summary

Taking responsibility for your fitness plays a crucial role in your success. Having this type of mindset helps you take control of your fitness and your life in general. Forget the gurus who tell you that it's somehow not your fault.

Most of our habits have become unconscious repetitions of the things that we've always been doing so start taking control of your fitness by looking at how you've set things up for yourself.

List down some of the things that can hinder you in your diet and training. Be brutally honest with the results, you've been having so far and start looking at the root causes behind your results. And if you've ever wondered whether your poor level of fitness might somehow be your fault, it is!

Action Steps:

1. Write down some of the things in fitness and health where you'd like to see some improvement.
If you don't know what that is yet, start looking at the results and work your way backwards. Be brutally honest here. I can't stress this enough since you're looking at some of the results of your unconscious behaviors and habits that have been built up over the years.

2. Ask yourself this: What habits have you created (or failed to create) that lead you to that specific result?

3. Ask yourself why you got there and write it down. Dig a little deeper and ask yourself why again. Keep on digging until you can no longer answer that question.

4. List down 2-3 small and easy-to-implement habits that you can create to solve your problem. Pick the one that you think will make the most impact for you.

Chapter 2

How To Keep Your Sanity On Your Fat Loss Journey

When you're starting out you'll often hear a lot of people emphasize the importance of going on a caloric deficit. That means you have to consume less than what your body burns off for a period of time. It sounds easy enough to do but let me ask you:

Do you often find yourself feeling deprived when you go on a caloric deficit? I'm willing to bet that you're probably asking yourself:

"How am I going to keep up with this without going insane?"

As one of my clients told me before:

"I want to lose weight but I love food too much! Can't figure out a way to stop eating them yet."

If this goes on long enough, do you start to feel guilt and loathe yourself if you slip up and start having a burger or a slice of cheesecake? Well, you're not alone. Dieters feel a lot of guilt when it comes to eating high calorie food.

Here's a typical scenario:

When you're just starting out on your journey to lose fat, you'll have a lot of fun during those first few weeks. You're doing something new and you're going to see results pretty quickly. You probably won't be surprised if you lost 2 or 3 lbs. a week.

But what happens after a month of being on a diet? Soon you'll find yourself getting bored or cutting back too much on your calories just to lose weight.

That's usually the part when most people start to deprive themselves of their favorite food. More often than not, they'll feel deprived because of their rigid diet. It's only a matter of time before they burn out as they start to plateau with the results.

In my case, my diet started to get more rigid after several weeks. Not being able to eat fattier cuts of meat or sweets made me miserable. Steaks, burgers and pizza somehow became "evil." I didn't eat out with my friends and the only semblance of a social life that I had was logging in to facebook or twitter.

Some of the gurus have popularized this trend of classifying food into good or bad. That's the reason why you'll hear a lot of dogma like don't eat white rice or anything that has wheat flour. In extreme cases, there's this phobia of fruit when it comes to fat loss. Believe it or not, some gurus or "doctors" would advice you to stop eating bananas so you can lose fat.

One of the biggest realizations for me was that keeping the quality of life is just as important in getting any kind of consistency in my diet and training. That means I had to have the types of food that I'd be happy with as well while staying within my maintenance of calories and fiber at the same time.

As a result, I made a list of the stuff that I couldn't last a week without. These include bread or white rice, burgers, pizza, ice cream , steak or fattier cuts of meat and chicken wings. All of these were non-negotiable for me. You can take this list further by making a list of non-negotiable food every month and a list for parties and special occasions.

Everyone has his list of non-negotiables and you can make changes to this list every month as you evaluate your fitness goals. Your list of non-negotiables will keep you from losing your sanity.

In the end, you'll find that there are only a few types of food that really fit that must-have criteria. And here's the fun part of it. You can plan when where and how much you can have them for the week. As a result, you'll end up appreciating them more without feeling guilty.

With that said, take a look at some of the calories of your favorite types of food as well as those that you're going to cut back on. This will give you a pretty good idea of the calories and macronutrients on them so you won't go overboard.

In my case, it was ice cream and fattier cuts of meat. I wouldn't last for a week if I didn't have any of these so I planned for them. It was one of those things that kept me sane throughout my journey because I had something to look forward to on the weekends.

Fitness is only good if you can maintain the kind of life that you want. Everybody has a list of the types of food that they can't live without. Write them down now and plan for them. Remember, if it's not sustainable in the long run, expect to gain back the weight that you've lost.

Summary

It's important for you to keep your quality of life when you're trying to lose fat. Forget about food dogma and list down some of your favorite foods as well as the portion sizes and their respective calories. It will help to keep you sane in the long run.

Action Steps:

1. Make a list of your non-negotiables every month with your calendar.

2. Visit websites that will help you count the calories of your food :

caloriecount.com,

myfitnesspal.com

fat secret.com

Figure out the number of calories per portion so you can include them in your diet every week.

Chapter 3

Focus on the Big Wins

When it comes to fat loss, people love to debate about the little things.

Should you go on a ketogenic diet? It can help you lose a lot of weight fast but then it has a lot of unwanted effects.

Should you eat carbohydrates at night? Do you really have to train early in the morning? How many meals per day?

Dieters often get overwhelmed with the amount of info that they're getting. And guess what most people do when they get overwhelmed with info?

They do absolutely nothing. It seems like their mind freezes up when confronted with more than a few choices. And that's not even the worst part of it.

Habits like this often go unnoticed. Years can go by and they'll often wonder what happened to all of those dieting secrets and info that they've been getting.

How come they're in no better shape now than when they first started out?

One of the best advices that I read about with this problem ironically comes from a guy who happens to eat a lot of junk food, Warren Buffet where he says:

"You only have to do a very few things right in your life so long as you don't do too many things wrong."

The thing is during those first few months you only need to make sure that you are at a caloric deficit and do it in such a way that you don't lose your sanity so you can maintain your consistency.

But what do most people do? They love to focus on ten different types of workouts and diets to help them get slimmer. And if they've gone bat shit crazy and neurotic, they'll do one different type of workout for each training day hoping that some kind of muscle confusion kicks in.

They'll keep on cutting back on their calories as well because they've read somewhere that carbohydrates or dairy are bad for fat loss. They start to develop this irrational fear of consuming carbohydrates.

And the bad news is they'll usually burn out within a few weeks. In fact, most people feel so emotionally drained with all of the workouts that they'll do the exact opposite. And I've seen this with some of my clients.

It seems as if something inside of them snaps. They'll rest a lot and eat a lot of sugary processed junk food. And if they were craving for a cheeseburger before, this time they want a 4 deck cheeseburger with fries and a tub of vanilla ice cream as their dip. And a couple weeks' worth of progress goes down the drain.

What they were really looking for is that magic bullet that will help them reach their weight loss goals faster. Most guys keep on looking for that little edge so they can lose weight faster.

The old way of doing things was to look at the next workout tip or fad diet that you get on youtube and try to implement it. Instead of looking for next workout fad or diet, look at what you're doing now. Look at the big picture and do an 80/20 on your diet and workouts. If you're not familiar with the 80/20 rule, it's a rule for focusing on the big things. That means 80% of your weight is the result of 20% of the things that you're doing with your diet and workouts.

Take a look at your diet. Where do the calories come from? If you're over x number of body fat percentage, there's a good chance that you have a lot of high calorie foods in there that you really don't want. Start creating the habit of taking those types of food out.

You can do that by starting a list of the high calorie foods that you can actually live without. These are usually the types of food that you tend to eat without even noticing that you're eating them.

The key to this whole exercise is to cut down on the things that you don't really want so you can save some of those calories for the things that you really do want in your life.

By the way, there should be no gray areas in some of the high-calorie foods that you want. If you sort of like something but you're not so sure, chances are good that you'll have to cut it from your diet.

The key here is to look at all of the things that you consume. Most guys make the mistake of looking at what they eat when they should be looking at the stuff that they're drinking as well.

There are a lot of high calorie drinks and sodas are loaded with them. Let's say you drink a can of coke every other day. In a week that adds up to about 556 calories. That's a lot of calories for something that does nothing for you. It's important to look at all of the calories that your body take in.

In my case, it was the potato chips and soda that I snacked on in between meals. In a week, they added up to almost 1000 calories.

Now take a look at your workouts, do you tend to do workouts that only focus on your abs? or biceps? Or butt? Or do you tend to stick to doing steady cardio like running? We'll talk more about this in the latter parts of the book.

Remember to start looking at the big picture of your diet and training and start optimizing things from there. Look at some of the things that you can easily eliminate from your diet and have the most impact for you in terms of calories. Take a good look at your workouts as well and see which types of workouts help you burn the most calories.

If you can do that, you'll be way ahead of the people who debate about whether or not they should eat carbohydrates at night or if they should eat steak or not.

Summary

Doing an 80/20 on your workouts helps you focus on the big picture of your fitness. Stop debating about minutiae and little fitness tips that won't affect your results that much. Instead, focus on what you can easily do right now that makes the biggest impact on your fitness. Doing this saves you a lot of time doing the important things and it helps you get things done without feeling overwhelmed.

Action Steps:

Take out a pen and paper and start answering these questions:

1. What are some of the key habits that you need to build right now that can give you massive results in terms of fat loss later?

2. How can you make it easy to implement them? Do you need to take small steps? Can you shorten the time that you perform these new habits so you can easily do them? How can you create a way to trigger these behaviors? Do you need an alarm a calendar or a timer?

3. What are some of the key habits that you need to eliminate?

4. How can you slowly eliminate these habits? Can you slowly eliminate these behaviors ? Can you replace them with healthier habits? What are some of your behaviors or events that trigger these behaviors?

Chapter 4

Knowing Where You Are

When you step on that weighing scale to monitor your progress, do you feel this dread starting to creep up?

Of course...we all have. A lot of people have this irrational fear of stepping on a weighing scale and looking at their weight. But let's dig a little deeper.

Why does stepping on that weighing scale bring so much dread and fear for you?

Is it the thought that you'll find out that you're very obese? Does that bring out your worst fears? Or is it the fact that you think you've made little to no progress when it comes to weight loss? By the way, using the weighing scale isn't a very accurate way of measuring your progress and we'll talk more about this in the latter parts of this chapter.

When I first started training some of my clients, I noticed a pattern about most people who are obese.
When you ask them about their weight or body fat percentage, 9 times out of 10 they'll tell you that they have no clue.

At first, I was surprised about this since it only takes a few seconds to step on a weighing scale. It made absolutely no sense at all.

It wasn't until a few weeks later that I figured this out. They had a situation that's very similar to people who had large amounts of credit card debt. They had this debilitating fear of opening up their monthly bills because they don't want to know the kind of trouble they're in.

In the case of fat loss, most of the guys don't want to see the amount of fat that has piled up for them over the years. It's a form of denial for them.

So how do you get over this fear of measuring your progress?

The way I see it, being obese and finding out about it is a lot like having a few bad grades in school. If you've ever performed poorly on a test, you felt this sense of dread as those test scores were being given. You probably didn't want to look at them and you felt devastated when you did.

Looking back at it now, you'll probably laugh at it because you realize that's not who you are. You probably don't even remember it that much anymore. The same thing goes for your body fat percentage or weight.

Your weight and body fat percentages are just tools to track your progress at a point in time and nothing more. When you look back on it years from now and see how far you've come, you'll probably laugh at how you use to dread them. They only seem worse than they really are. When you keep things in perspective, you'll realize that where you are now isn't as important as where you're going.

So how do you measure your progress? The weighing scale is the most common method out there but using that alone isn't very accurate in measuring your progress. The same goes for the BMI, which measures your height and weight.

Here's why:
Your weight has two components-the weight that comes from fat and the weight that comes from the rest of your body. The weighing scale doesn't take that into account. It simply measures your weight.

You can have two people with the same height and the same weight and they can look completely different from each other. An obese guy with a height of 6'0 can have a weight of 170 lb but so can a muscular guy of the same height.

With that said, I'd like to invite you to change the way you measure your fitness from looking at your weight alone to focusing on improving your body composition as well by looking at the amount of fat in your body. Knowing your body composition paints an accurate picture of your progress.

There are two ways for you to monitor your body composition. The easiest way is to buy a tape measure and take your measurements first thing in the morning before you have your meals. That will give you a pretty good idea about your body composition. Using the tape measure gives you a pretty good idea of your progress.

The second way of measuring your body composition is to look at your body fat percentage. You'll get a pretty accurate picture of how someone looks if you know their body fat percentage regardless of their height or weight.

You can use a caliper, bio-electric impedance machine, or use a fat percentage calculator on the internet. Of these 3, the first one is the most accurate but you need to be very well trained and it takes too long. The second one isn't very accurate and it's the most expensive. I recommend you use the last one. All you need to do is get your weight and waist measurements as well as your height and input the values on some of these websites:

http://www.calculator.net/army-body-fat-calculator.html

http://home.fuse.net/clymer/bmi/

And here's the biggest benefit that you can get from acquiring this habit:

You'll be able to avoid unnecessary fat loss plateaus that stalls the progress of most guys. Everyone who fails to measure their progress the right way will almost always encounter unnecessary plateaus in their journey towards fat loss.

The reason for that is simple. As you start to lose weight, your body adapts to what you've been doing and sooner or later, you'll have to adapt with your diet and training as well. When you measure your progress, you can clearly see the need for you to adapt your diet and training to your new body fat percentage and weight.

This tool can save you weeks of worry and frustration.

One of the biggest mistakes that most beginners make is to take these measurements once they've had their meals. I recommend you take these measurements when you wake up. This is the only way that you can be consistent with your measurements.

Summary

Knowing how to measure your progress plays a crucial role in fat loss. Building this habit may seem intimidating at first but they're just tools to help you keep track of where you are. Learn how to measure your body fat percentage will give you an edge over using the weighing scale alone because it gives you a very good estimate of your body composition.

If you prefer an easier method of measuring your body composition, the tape measure makes for an excellent tool. You can take this a bit further by taking your waist measurement, weight and height to get your body fat percentage from several websites. Building this habit will give you consistency and keep you from having those fat loss plateaus.

Action Steps:

1. Buy a tape measure and a weighing scale. You can easily purchase them online through Amazon or any other store.

2. Set a date on Google calendar or your manual calendar for you to measure your progress. Make sure you set this every 2-4 weeks and take your measurements when you wake up before you consume anything.

3. Start taking your waist measurement and your weight.

4. Input these on either of these websites:

http://www.calculator.net/army-body-fat-calculator.html

http://home.fuse.net/clymer/bmi/

Chapter 5

The Best Bodyweight Exercise

One question that I often get asked by some of my busy clients is: What is the best bang for my buck exercise? For the small period of time that I have in the gym what can I do?

One of the best exercises that you can do is the pull-up. If you can only do one exercise, make it the pull-up or chin-up. The pull-up/chin-up easily ranks as the best bodyweight exercise. Not only that, the pull-up is also considered as the king of the upper-body exercises.

In fact, you can literally design an entire workout program with different variations of the pull-up/chin-up. Depending on how much time you have, you can go extreme or do several sets of them. Once you start getting the hang of it, I guarantee that you will have a more athletic looking body.

Our ancestors have been doing this since the dawn of mankind and there's no reason why we can't do the same. We've been climbing up trees or cliffs by pulling our bodies up. It's basically what we've been doing to survive.

So what's the difference between a pull-up and a chin-up?

It all boils down to hand-position. With the chin up, you have your palms facing toward you while you have your palms facing away from you on the pull-up.

If you spend time doing pull-ups, I can guarantee that you'll see the difference in your physique. No bodyweight exercise builds up your upper body quite like the pull-up. If you do the pull-up, you emphasize the back muscles such as your lats (latisimuss dorsi muscle). With the chin-up, you get to focus more on your biceps.

Both types of exercises also work on your back and core stabilizing muscles. These muscles play a crucial role as you start lifting heavier weights.

Now, you're probably thinking to yourself:

"What? Pull-ups? Are you nuts? I can't even do one single repetition of that exercise! I don't want to go to the gym and embarrass myself."

That's the thing about pull-ups and chin-ups. Nothing inspires awe and fear among beginners than the pull-up. Pull-ups are the gold standard of fitness tests.

But the thing is you're not alone. In fact, you'll see some guys who have been in the gym for years, who can't do more than 1 or 2 pull-ups. In a few moments, I'll show you how I was able to get that first rep and started increasing my repetitions from there.

When I first encountered the pull-up, I already knew how hard it was going to be. Waiting for my turn in gym class, I had this fear of not being able to make one repetition. Almost every other kid got at least 1 rep and I figured if I could do one, I'll save myself the embarrassment. As soon as it was my turn, I started using momentum by jumping so I could get just one rep in.

Sadly, the PE teacher, who looked like a cross between Chyna the female wrestler and Jillian Michaels was having none of it. I had to start from a dead hang and I haven't tried to perform the same exercise for the next few years for fear of embarrassment.

It wasn't until almost a decade later that I realized that I wasn't alone. Even some of the veteran guy in the gym found pull-ups hard. So I started focusing on getting just one single rep.

I started looking at how I can get to that one single rep and there are two ways you can gain enough strength to get one pull-up. The first one is the assisted pull-up. As you're hanging from the bar, your foot is supported by a chair and you can push off the chair to get some momentum as you pull yourself up.

Another way is to do negative pull-ups. Negative pull-ups are pull-ups done in reverse where you start by jumping off to the final position with your chin on the bar and slowly lower yourself. This is where you descend as slowly as possible. Once you can slow down your rate of descent to around 5-6 seconds, you'll be strong enough to do one single rep.

What I discovered was that it was better to combine both methods in a single repetition. I started using the assisted pull-up on the way up and letting go of the foot supporting my weight and using the negative pull-up on the way down. This habit is perfect for those who can't perform a single repetition and I found that within 2-3 weeks I could do a few reps without any kind of assistance.

Now you're probably wondering whether you should do the pull-up or the chin-up. If you're still starting out, I recommend you go for the chin-up so you can make it easier for yourself to have that one good rep.

Most beginners make the mistake of positioning their hands too far apart. Try to keep your hands shoulder-width apart. This helps you prevent any unnecessary injuries and it gives you a good mechanical advantage to make it easy for you to perform a single rep. You can experiment with the types of grip and distance later on.

In general, the more advance you get, the more distance you can have in between your hands. This gives you less of a mechanical advantage and it works on your targeted muscles more.

In case you're wondering whether the pull-up or the chin-up is better than the other, remember what I told you about going for the big wins instead of debating about minutiae? Frankly, I recommend doing both types of exercises.

For a more advanced version of the pull-up, you can do around the world pull-ups. This is the type of pull-up where you move your torso to one side as you move up and once you reach the peak of the pull-up, you move your torso to the other side and move down slowly. This helps to develop the bicep area of your muscles.

Summary

The pull-up is the best body weight and upper body exercise out there. With that said it can be one of the more challenging types of exercises for beginners but the results are more than worth it. A lot of beginners are intimidated with the pull-up or chin-up because they can't perform a single repetition yet. The key to all of this is to use assisted pull-ups and negative pull-ups in combination to shorten the amount of time that you can start doing pull-ups. The pull-up has a lot of variations and they work on the different parts of the body.

Action Steps:

1. Buy one of those pull-up bars that are sold in Amazon or you can go to the gym.

2. Set an alarm on your calendar for 2 days/ week where you can do these pull-ups or set a date on your manual calendar.

3. Have a chair or bench that you could set your foot on to support you on your way up and slowly release your support foot on your descent. That counts as 1 repetition

4. Do 1 set of 5-7 repetitions.

5. Gradually increase your number of sets to 3-4 sets.

Chapter 6

Using The Best Types of Exercises for Fat Loss

Isn't it interesting how we claim that we want to burn more fat —and we really do want to- but if we took a closer look at our workouts, we haven't really burned a lot of calories at all.

Now some of that may be due to the lack of good information out there and some of it may be due to applying the information at the wrong time. There are a lot of magazines that sell you on how to get bigger biceps, triceps and abs. but most of the stuff that you read on magazines don't give you the foundational workouts that are necessary.

In a few moments, I'll show you how to workout less and burn more calories with weights.

One of the biggest mistakes that most beginners make when they're just starting out is that they tend to follow the advice given in fitness magazines about targeting a specific body part. Most of the time they'll tell you to do isolation exercises like bicep curls or abdominal crunches.

But what happens after that? If you've ever tried doing one of those workouts in fitness magazines, you'll find that a lot of them won't really work for you. Most of these types of titles usually have something to the effect of "Get great abs for only 7 min. a day."

It makes for a catchy title but 99% of the time it gives you lousy results. You'll end up confused and frustrated as hell because you're doing everything that you can and you won't have the results to show for it.

The truth is that training programs like these are usually more suited for intermediate to advanced trainees or lifters.

I could recall a time when I did 7 or 8 of these exercises that use machines and I had almost nothing to show for it. I was confused as hell and I actually wondered if there was something wrong with me.

It was probably one of the most frustrating parts about losing weight because I've been consistent with my training and I wasn't seeing any kind of improvement. If you've ever seen one of those cartoon shows where the bad guy runs into a brick wall after chasing his prey around for hours, that's what it feels like.

What most people need when they're starting out are the basic compound (multi-joint) lifts or exercises to get them to burn more calories.

Think about it for a second.

What do you think burns more calories? The traditional bicep curl or the chin up? When you look at it, your body does more work with the latter simply because more joints are involved. The more joints you involve, the more muscles get to work. As a result, you get to lift or put more resistance or weight in your exercises.

In his book the Truth About Six Pack Abs Mike Geary shows the importance of having full body workouts. He shows that your body tends to do more work when it does compound lifts.

Now I know that some people will be upset that I'm talking about math when explaining this concept but hear me out for a second.

Work =force x distance

Your limbs will cover more distance when multiple joints are involved. In contrast with the bicep curl, the only distance covered is that of the forearms rotating. You also have the potential to exert more force as you lift heavier weights with multiple joints involved.

The last part is crucial as it allows you to progress faster. I can't emphasize the importance of doing multi-joint exercises. If you fail to set up your training to include multi-joint exercises, be prepared for the head-scratching frustration that comes your way. It's a lot worse than taking that money that you use for the gym and tearing it up. At least you'll have saved yourself some time.

A research from Applied Physiology Nutrition and Metabolism also shows that when single joint exercises are added to multi-joint exercises for untrained individuals, there's no significant difference in muscle size and strength.[2]

Their experiment examined 29 untrained young men, who participated in a 10-week exercise program. They were divided randomly into 2 groups. The first group performed only multi-joint exercises while the second group performed multi-joint exercises while adding some single joint exercises as well.

---

[2] P. Gentil, *Effect of Adding Single-Joint Exercises to Multi-Joint Exercise Training Program on Strength and Hypertrophy on Untrained Subjects* (Applied Physiology Nutrition and Metabolism, 2013).

Although both groups showed a significant increase in strength and muscle thickness, they had no differences in terms of strength and size improvements.

When you're starting out, focus on the multi-joint exercises first. You can add the single joint exercises after a month or two.

With that said, it's time to create your habit of multi-joint training. And one of the best ways to do that is to use the compound lifts. This habit will help you burn calories in less time.

Summary

There has always been this trend of emphasizing your workouts on a single body part. These types of workouts don't burn enough calories for the beginner to even justify his time in the gym. In fact, most if not all of these workouts should be reserved for the intermediate lifters.

To burn more calories for your workouts focus on the compound movements where more joints are involved for every type of exercise. This helps you to burn 3-4 times more calories than the single joint workout.

It's important to build the habit of having compound lifts when you're starting out. If you don't add those lifts now, you'll wander around trying different isolation exercises and probably never land on something that works.

Action Steps

1. Set your alarm and calendar for the next day

2. Get all of your workout gear ready the night before you workout

3. Perform the workouts on alternate days
Keep track of your progress by recording it in a notebook

Workout A

Chin-up   2 sets of 5-9 repetitions

Pushups 4 sets of 8 repetitions

Deadlifts 4 sets of 8 repetitions

Workout B

Pull-ups 2 sets of 5-9 repetitions

Goblet Squat 4sets of 8 repetitions

Barbell Rows 4 sets of 8 repetitions

Chapter 7

The Most Crucial Type of Training for Getting Leaner and Stronger

I've got a question for you. Do you have running or cardio as your main workout?

Have you ever thought to yourself that you'll probably just skip the weights? You're probably scared that you might get too bulky if you started doing them. You're probably telling yourself that you just want "to look lean and athletic."

Have you always wanted to go to the gym but you get nervous and end up not going because the other guys might laugh at you? Or maybe you think that it's too much work to get that athletic look.

By the way, it's not exactly fun to feel self-conscious when you're lifting weights in the gym and thinking that everyone's just looking at you and waiting for you to fail. I'm sure that most people would rather skip the weights and keep doing the things that they've been doing before.

When I was starting out, I ran 3-4 times a week thinking that it would help me get 6 pack abs. I had around 7-8 single-joint exercises and some ab workouts for 3-4 times a week. Now you can probably guess what happened after a few months.

I had zero results. Running so many times a week and doing isolation exercises was exhausting and after seeing those results, I was one pissed off dude.

Now I know that most women are scared of weights because they're afraid of getting bulky. But ironically, I got started with strength training when I got some advice from a female personal trainer.

Several years ago, I could remember this statuesque personal trainer asking me if I've been doing any strength training. She suggested some of the basic moves but I was having none of it. In my head, I was thinking to myself:

"and what do you know about working out and losing fat lady?"

I actually thought that I knew more about training than the personal trainer based on my 21-year-old naiveté. For me, there was no way she was teaching me anything about losing fat.

As a result, I skipped one of the most crucial aspects to losing fat- increasing and maintaining my lean body mass. It wasn't more than a couple months later when I realized how right she was. I finally decided to give it a shot and I was working out less and seeing better results.

This is probably the part where I should tell you to check your ego at the front door. Being stubborn, ignorant and egotistic always lead to disaster. You'll be surprised at how effective these 3 things are in stalling your progress.

You've probably seen people compare the athletic look of sprinters with that of the marathoners. A lot of people think that comes from sprinting.

But the truth is that most of that look comes from good old fashioned strength training. In a typical week, sprinters will do 3-4 sessions of strength training. That's a whole lot more than your average marathoner.

Strength training helps you increase your muscle mass and gives you that athletic look.

To quote one of the best strength coaches Mark Rippetoe: "That's going to have a huge impact on how you look and how strong you are."

Have you ever seen guys and girls have the skinny-fat condition? That's the kind of body where there's fat concentrated on the belly, butt and thighs and the rest of the body looks skinny.

Have you ever been skinny fat yourself? One of the secrets to getting rid of that condition is to start building up your lean body mass.

The amount of lean muscle mass that you have dictates your resting metabolic rate. The more lean body mass you have, the more calories you'll need. And that's good news for those who don't want to starve while trying to get six pack abs. In the end, you'll look athletic instead of skinny fat.

I know that some women still feel uncomfortable with weights because they don't want the female bodybuilder's physique.

But let me tell you those results came after years of lifting very heavy weights and they've been progressing very consistently. It takes a lot of time to build the bodybuilder's physique and this is especially true for females. Those results didn't happen by accident and they certainly didn't happen overnight where they woke up one day and got muscular all of a sudden.

And if you're still in doubt, take a look at those Victoria's Secret Models. I can guarantee you this, they didn't get that kind of physique by running alone. To achieve that kind of physique, they had to do some form of strength training consistently.

There's a good reason why strength training programs have been around for a long time. They work very well in terms of improving how your body functions and how you'll look in the end. They don't take a lot of time and more importantly, they don't require a thousand moves to get one workout done. Take a look at one of the workouts below and see if you'd rather be doing those muscle confusion types of exercises or strength training. I can guarantee you the latter will give you better results in less time.

Summary

Strength training helps you achieve that athletic physique. If you've ever compared the physique of sprinters and marathoners, you'll notice the difference. The physique of sprinters largely comes from the fact that they do 3-4 times of strength training per week. Strength training also helps to keep you from having that skinny-fat problem with your physique and contrary to popular belief, it helps women look better.

Action Steps:

1. Set your alarm and calendar for the next day

2. Get all of your workout gear ready the night before you workout

3. Perform the workouts on alternate days

Workout A

Chin up / assisted chin up 4 sets of 5 repetitions

Rows 3 sets of 5 repetitions

Deadlift 3 sets of 5 repetitions

Workout B

Front Squat 4 sets of 5 repetitions

Military Press 3 sets of 5 repetitions

Bench Press 3 sets of 5 repetitions

4. Keep track of your progress by recording it in a notebook or Excel.

Chapter 8

Cardio That Helps You Burn More Fat

Do you always feel like you have no time to do your cardio exercise? If you're busy working throughout the day and doing chores at night, chances are good that you'll only have less than 30 min. to workout.

So what type of cardio helps you get the most bang for your buck in transforming your physique?

One of the best ways is high intensity interval training or HIIT as they call it.

HIIT burns more calories on a given period of time compared to steady state cardio and the intensity required from HIIT will deplete the glycogen (carbohydrates stores as energy) in your muscles very quickly. Once your glycogen stores are depleted, your body starts to look at fat as its fuel.

Here's the great thing about HIIT. There's a popular research called the Tremblay study where researchers did comparisons of skin-fold tests between those who did HIIT and those who did steady state cardio. They found that those who did HIIT lost 3 times as much fat based on the skin-fold test for 1/3 of the time invested. [3]

---

[3] Angelo Tremblay, *Impact of Exercise Intensity on Body Fatness and Skeletal Muscle Metabolism* (Metabolism , 1994).

Does this mean that steady state cardio is useless? I wrote an article about that on my blog. You can check it out:

http://surewaytofitness.com/2014/11/08/the-honest-truth-about-steady-state-cardio-high-intensity-interval-training/

You have several choices when it comes to doing interval training. Your main goal however is to avoid injuries that usually result from doing things too fast too soon.

Summary

HIIT is an excellent way of helping you transform your physique and it helps you save a lot of time. It provides the most bang for your buck when it comes to doing cardio. It also helps you to achieve fat loss faster than the regular type of steady cardio. There are different types of interval training with varying intensities and you can start doing the easiest one first and move your way up. Find a way to incorporate these workouts to your daily habit.

Here are some of the habits that you can build. Pick one and do this for a month or two.

Fartlek training:

20-30 minutes

By far the easiest form of interval training, fartlek was invented by the Swedish. It literally means speed play. In this type of training, you increase the intensity of the exercise whenever you want.

Keys to Fartlek:
Fartlek is a very unstructured form of HIIT and you can increase the speed and pace as you wish. Slowly build up your speed and make sure you warm up to prevent injuries.

Action Steps:
1. Set your alarm on your Google calendar or do this manual with your alarm clock and calendar.
2. Jog for 2-3 min. and increase your intensity for 20-40 sec.
3. Go back to jogging and increase the intensity when you feel like it.
4. Do this for the next 10 min. of your jog.

5. For the next 10 min. start doing 10-15 sec. sprints for every 2 min. of jogging.

Tabata

Total time 14-16 min.

The tabata protocols was one of the most well-researched forms of HIIT. The original protocol used bikes as they're less likely to cause injury. You can do the same for running or even body weight training exercises.

The tabata protocols will take a toll on your body so make sure to warm up first to prevent injuries. Do this twice per week:

Steps:

1. Set your alarm on your Google calendar or do this manual with your alarm clock and calendar.

2. Warm up for 10 min.

3. 3. Go hard for 20 sec. of 8 rounds of all our effort.

4. Rest for 10 sec in between rounds.

Chapter 9

The Crucial Habit To Build Your Own Diet

I'd like to address one problem that's very common for dieters who are just starting out.

There's a situation where most people who are starting out use their emotions to sabotage themselves when they're setting up their diet.

This fear of setting up your diet can become a habit and most books will skirt around the issue by telling you that calories are somehow an inaccurate way of knowing how much you're consuming.

Let me ask you this:

Have you ever thought about counting your calories and told yourself not to bother because you couldn't do them accurately anyway?

Or maybe you didn't figure out how many calories, protein and fat you should be consuming because you figured that you'd waste too much time trying to figure it out?

There are a lot of crazy diets out there and around 90% of them probably won't work very well for you.

And let me ask you this:
If you go through with that restrictive diet and you happen to get invited to a party where that slice of steak is right in front of you, what are you going to do about it?

Chances are you're going to gorge yourself because you couldn't resist what's in front of you or you'll end up trying to ignore the damned thing. In short you're going to use that willpower to resist having your favorite food.

And you might even succeed, but for how long? Can you keep that up for a week? A few months?

Most people have this debilitating fear of setting up their diet because they think it's too complicated and what happens is that they usually end up going through a diet that deprives of them what they actually want to eat.

One of the biggest mistakes that I see most guys make is not setting up their calories. Not knowing how many calories and macronutrients you have to consume is a lot like going to a new city without a map.

Sure you can avoid high calorie foods and still lose weight but as the months go by it's going to get harder for you to lose fat.

Now some people may hate counting calories and math in general. But here's the thing, setting up your calories takes less than 5 min. of your time.

Now there are some of you who will say that you don't need to count calories. All you need to do is eat clean because 100 calories of quinoa isn't the same as 100 calories of sugar.

To an extent that's true. You can lose weight and have better long term healthy when you eat clean. But can you keep your sanity? Most guys I know would go nuts if you deprive them of burgers and pizza.

And besides, trying to maintain your caloric levels would mean that you'd have to eat clean most of the time anyway.

Think of counting your maintenance calories as having a roadmap in your journey to losing fat. You'll have the peace of mind knowing that you won't get lost along the way.

On the other hand, look at eating clean as you simply avoiding the dark alleys and corners of a city. You can definitely do that but sooner or later you'll get lost, wander around and keep doing the same thing. And you're going to ask yourself why you're getting nowhere with your diet.

And while it's true that measuring calories is a crude way of measuring energy since you're basically looking at how much energy it takes to burn off the food, it's a heck of a lot better than having no clue at all.

Sooner or later your weight will pretty much be a reflection of the amount of macronutrients and calories that you took in and out. You can't get around that fact unless you're on drugs.

One more thing, do you notice how people tend to frown on pizza and burgers when they're on a diet? It seems as if there's this category of food that's downright evil. Nine times out of ten, the people who do this can't be bothered to count their calories. Think about it. Pizza and burgers are nothing more than a mix of bread, cheese, tomato and beef. They're basically made of stuff that you wouldn't consider as bad or evil in the first place.

The problem comes from the fact that classifying food as good or bad is just a shorthand for most dieters to cut back on their calories. Doing that will help you initially but in the long run, you'll encounter a lot of problems with your diet when it stops working.

One of the biggest mistakes that most dieters make is to base their computations on their current weight. This presents a lot of problems for them as they try to eat less than their maintenance calories- a figure which keeps on changing over time.

The secret to setting up your diet is to base your caloric intake on your target bodyweight instead of simply looking at your current maintenance calories.

If you weigh 170 lbs. and you want to get lean at 160, you have to eat like a 160 lb. man. Alan Aragon, one of the best nutritionists in the industry was one of the first to use this type of computation. Most of the computations below are based on his research.

Summary

A lot of dieters have issues with setting up the diet. Most of the main reasons include not being able to do it accurately and not having enough time. Counting the calories that you'll need helps you avoid unnecessary fat loss plateaus. It also helps you consume the types of food that you want instead of avoiding them altogether because you think it's junk.

If you make it a habit to set up your diet every few weeks or every month, you'll have a pretty clear roadmap to your success in losing fat. The key to all of this is to make sure that you base your maintenance on your target body weight instead of using your current weight.

Here's how you can build the habit:

Step 1 Setting up your triggers
Set up your Google calendar and alarm for the first day of each month

Step 2 Set your targeted weight
Find your ideal weight

Step 3 Computing for your daily caloric expenditure

Target Weight x (8 to 11 calories per lb. + number of training hours per week)= total daily caloric expenditure

The multiplier is based on gender and your level of activity.

8-sedentary women

9-active women and sedentary men

10- very active women and active men

11- very active men

Step 4 Compute for your protein requirements

Total fat mass= total weight x body fat percentage

Lean body mass= total weight- total fat mass

0.8 to 1 gram / lb. x lean body mass = Total Protein in grams

Protein in grams x 4 calories per gram of protein= Total Number of Calories for Protein

Step 5 Compute for fat requirements

Target bodyweight x .5 gram per lb. = Total fat in grams

Total fat in grams x 9 calories per gram of fat = Total Number of Calories for Fat

Step 6 Compute for carbohydrate requirements

Total Daily Caloric Expenditure- Total Number of Calories from Fat – Total Number of Calories from Protein = Total Number of calories from Carbohydrates

Step 7 Maintenance

After setting up your calories, set an alarm on your calendar for the next couple of sessions where you'll be doing this computation as your goals change. You can do this every 2 or 3 months or you can simply stick to your plan if you prefer.

Author's Note:

You can have different computations for your total daily caloric expenditure. Some people prefer using lean body mass to compute for the figures however building the habit of computing for you calories is more important at this stage. With that said, the calculations above are the easiest way to do these calculations and it's perfect for those who are starting out.

Chapter 10 How to Estimate Your Calories

Now you're probably asking how you're going to count your calories accurately after you've set up your diet. In a few moments, I'll show you how you can learn how to estimate them pretty accurately.

One of the big problems that most dieters encounter is this fear of being inaccurate when they're counting their calories.

Have you ever had that feeling that you're not counting your calories accurately?

Or thought to yourself:
"What's the point of counting calories? That only takes the fun away from eating?"

I'd like to invite you to see it from a different perspective. If you know how to estimate your calories, doesn't that free up your mind from the guilt of consuming your favorite food?

One of the biggest reasons why most guys fail when they're trying to lose fat is that they almost always underestimate the calories they've been consuming. This usually leads to fat loss plateaus.

More often than not it discourages the dieter from pursuing his long term goals of sustained fat loss. Imagine spending a few weeks or months wondering why you're not making any kind of progress with your diet.

If you've ever had fat loss plateaus, chances are good that it's about your diet. If you've already reset your calories and taken your new body fat percentage and weight into account, there's a big chance you're underestimating your calories.

Now you're probably thinking that there's no way you can be so precise with counting your calories just by looking at the food in front of you. And I've got some good news for you. Nobody does!

Even the professional bodybuilders can't give precise estimates of the calories they're consuming by simply looking at their food. You only need to get a pretty good estimate of the calories that you're consuming so you can eat your food without feeling guilty.

With that said, the only way that you can be precise with counting your calories is to use a food scale and acquiring the skill of estimating your calories will be well worth your time.

So here's how you can learn the habit of estimating your calories. This will take about 20 min. of your time.

After doing this for a few days a week, you'll have a pretty good feel as to how many calories you're consuming.

You can use this on your cheat days or when you're eating out. Remember to overestimate your calories so you won't go overboard.

Keep in mind that you're never going to be completely accurate when you're counting your calories. But having a good estimate will help you go a long way on your diet as you'll have a good idea of the amount of calories you're taking in.

Summary

Most dieters have this idea that counting your calories will keep them from enjoying their diet. This couldn't be further from the truth. Learning how to estimate your calories allows you to enjoy your food without the guilt. Nobody can do this very accurately without the use of a weighing scale so take the time to practice this habit. Soon you'll have a pretty good idea how many calories you're consuming. Remember to overestimate the calories you're consuming when you're eating out as well.

Action Steps:

1. Buy a weighing scale for your food on Amazon or any other website.
2. Prepare your measuring cups, spoons and weighing scales and set an alarm on your Google calendar.
3. Weigh the meat and look up the calories in one of those fitness websites.
Take a slice and weigh it again. Now look up the total number of calories.
4. Fill a cup of your favorite carbohydrates and put it on your plate. Go and look it up on the website.
5. Now take 1 tbsp. of oil that you normally use and pour it over the meat and look up the amount of calories in the website.

Chapter 11

How To Keep Your Hormone Levels From Slowing Down Your Fat Loss On A Diet

Here's one of the most common questions that I often get asked about:

"Adam, you say you can help people lose fat but how do you do it without driving people insane? I love food too much and I want carbohydrates. Lots of it! I can't lose fat with carbohydrates right?"

With the Ketogenic and Paleo dieting craze, people are starting to have this irrational fear of getting fat by ingesting some carbohydrates.

It's true that ketogenic diets (or paleo) can help you lose a lot of weight initially because they have a lot of similarities with your body's reaction to starvation. But what's more likely to happen is that most people go off on the diet because they can't live with the low carbohydrate consumption.

What if I told you there's a way around that that would help you lose fat better. In a few moments, I'll show you how you can lose fat, keep your sanity and grow muscle at the same time.

People used to look at dieting imply as having less calories going in their bodies and more calories going out. While it's a useful way of looking at fat loss, there's one key ingredient that's missing- managing your hormones. Managing your hormones will help you make the most out of your diet and keep you from getting frustrated with having fat loss plateaus.

Your hormones dictate the types of nutrients that your body will use. It largely dictates how much fat you get to lose and keep. You should learn how to manage your hormones while you're on a diet to keep your fat loss from slowing down to a crawl.

With that said, do note that the interaction between your hormones is a complicated process. In fact there's more than enough information out there to make your head spin so I'll get straight to the point. Your hormones are neither good nor evil. People have this tendency to classify different hormones as good or bad.

They exist simply to help your body survive and thrive. It doesn't care about your six pack abs or your body composition. In this chapter, we'll cover some of the hormones that can help and hinder you from losing fat as well as how to manage them.

One of the most important things that you can do to achieve the goal of sustained fat loss is to learn how to manage your insulin levels.

Insulin is the main hormone that influences fat loss. What's more is that it affects the levels of your other hormones that lead to fat loss.

It is better known as the storage hormone as it takes the nutrients in your blood stream and into the storage depots.

Fatty acids for instance get stored in fat tissue aka adipose tissue. Sugar on the other hand gets stored as muscle glycogen and the excess gets converted into fat where it gets stored in adipose tissue. Insulin's main job is to help your body grow and store more energy for its survival. In fact, Insulin does a better job of helping your muscles grow compared to growth hormone.

The bad news is that it really doesn't care how your body grows. You can have lots of muscle and a lot of fat as well.

Remember, insulin doesn't care about your six pack abs because it has no value in terms of survival.

One of Insulin's main advantages include the formation of glycogen, which is sugar turned into energy for your muscles instead of being converted into fat as well as giving you energy for your intense workouts.

According to Brandon Carter, a fitness model and personal trainer, it helps move the proteins in the form of branch chain amino acids to your muscle cells. It activates the ribosomes that help to synthesize the protein. This helps to increase muscle size and prevents the breakdown of your muscles. [4]

On the other hand, it increases the formation of fatty acids in your liver, which can be burned off if you lack carbohydrates (muscle glycogen) or stored as body fat.

It also shifts the metabolism of the nutrients in your body. Instead of burning off fat, it utilizes carbohydrates instead.

It also inhibits HSL, which is responsible for the breakdown of the fat molecules.[5]

_____

[4] Brandon Carter, *Ultimate Cuts* (B & B Sports Nutrition ,2014).

[5] Ibid

Another hormone that helps you burn off more fat is Leptin. Leptin controls a number of metabolic functions in your body that lead to fat loss. Ironically, Leptin comes from your fat cells. And the less fat you have, the less Leptin you'll produce. Eating below your caloric maintenance after a few days leads to a drop in your leptin levels and it will slow down the rate of fat loss.

With that said about your hormones, you will then need to manage your insulin levels so you can build lean muscle mass, which leads to a higher resting metabolism. At the same time you want to get them to lower levels to help you burn off fat.

To do that you need a strategic cyclical diet where you can time your nutrients to increase your insulin levels to build and keep your muscle mass and drop them to lower levels to help you lose fat.

When I first learned about this stuff, I used a form of zigzag diet to keep myself from going crazy. I'd have 4-5 days of caloric deficit and 2 days of eating a little bit more than usual. The 2 day break in this diet helped my hormones return back to normal levels after several days of dieting.

In his book titles, Holy Grail Body Transformation, Tom Venuto makes an excellent point of having 3 days of caloric deficit and 1 day of being at maintenance and having a normal meal. At the same time you want most of your carbohydrates after the workouts to maximize muscle growth. [6]

This type of diet makes it easier for you to go on a diet while keeping your hormones at normal levels at the same period of time.

Summary

Our bodies have evolved to store fat as a means of being able to store and use energy efficiently. Your hormones such as Insulin and leptin have a crucial role in dictating how much fat you'll burn off. Learn how to manage them on your diet. You can do this by going through a cyclical diet of having 3 days on a deficit and 1 day of eating a little more. Make sure that you're on a caloric deficit for the entire week. If you do these things, you will help you bring your hormones back to normal levels so you can lose fat faster.

---

[6] Tom Venuto, *Holy Grail Body Transformation* (Fitness Renaissance LLC, 2010).

Action Steps:

1. Set an alarm on your Google Calendar or App. on your off days so you can do groceries and prepare your food for the week ahead.
2. Buy foods that you can readily eat such as lettuce, canned chicken breast or tuna or canned garbanzo beans.
3. You can bring these types of food to work easily for the next 5 days.
4. Go on a normal diet for 1-2 days after your first 5 days of dieting.

Note:

You can start the habit of doing your groceries and cooking and repacking your food later. You can add more variety but the key here is to have easy wins so you can start building momentum for your diet.

Stacking Your Habits One At A Time

I want to end this book with the emphasis on building your habits. As much as I'd like you to implement all of the habits outlined in this book immediately, that's unrealistic at best and disastrous at worst.

That you read and understood all of the theory and parts of this book isn't the most important thing. The crucial part is to take action until these habits become a part of who you are. Start with one habit and slowly stack them together as you progress.

There's that old saying " I hear I forget. I see. I remember. I do. I understand." That pretty much sums up what this book is all about.

Debating about minutiae on how to optimize your workouts and looking for that next weird tip will not help you get the results that you want. Think about it, How many people do you know who got six pack abs with the weird tips?

If you stay consistent with your new habits and you keep on progressing on your workouts and diet, I guarantee that you'll be much further ahead of the people looking for the next shortcut.

Remember that you can lose weight quickly (I'm talking about months here) but you can't lose weight quickly and easily unless you're on drugs or you've had a surgical operation.

A lot of people believe in the hype and marketing but remember that our bodies aren't wired to gain a lot of muscle and lose fat. It takes dedication and being systematic about your approach to fitness to achieve those results.

Let's summarize some of the main ideas in this book

1. Having the right mindset such as taking responsibility, being committed and focused on the crucial things is important.

2. Focus on the habit of doing the exercises that help you burn off more calories instead of worrying about a single body part.

3. Your diet is a crucial part of losing fat. Learn how to build the habit of taking in calories that help you maintain the optimal levels for your hormones. They will help you lose fat faster. Learn the skill of estimating your calories and knowing your daily maintenance.

For more information how to lose fat check out my blog.

You'll get lots of info on how to lose fat and you can get a **free copy** of my mini-course and fat-loss newsletters at www.surewaytofitness.com.

If you enjoyed this book, please leave a 5 star review for us as well. If you didn't please let us know at adambritonlee@gmail.com

If you have any questions, comments or feedback, please let me know as well. I try to answer all of the questions personally or in my mailbag and I read all of them personally.

The 11 Effective Fat Loss Habits

By Adam Briton Lee

SWTF Press
First Edition, 2014

before any new diet,
exercise or other health program.

www.ingramcontent.com/pod-product-compliance
Lightning Source LLC
Chambersburg PA
CBHW062015280526
45787CB00005B/2105